SO YOU'RE THINKING
ABOUT **KIDNEY**
TRANSPLANTATION

DR. MARK K. WEDEL, MD, FACP

SO YOU'RE THINKING ABOUT **KIDNEY** **TRANSPLANTATION**

A Patient and Family's Guide

With an Introduction by former NFL running back **John Brockington**

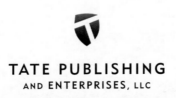

TATE PUBLISHING
AND **ENTERPRISES**, LLC

Published by Tate Publishing & Enterprises, LLC
127 E. Trade Center Terrace | Mustang, Oklahoma 73064 USA
1.888.361.9473 | www.tatepublishing.com

Tate Publishing is committed to excellence in the publishing industry. The company reflects the philosophy established by the founders, based on Psalm 68:11,
"The Lord gave the word and great was the company of those who published it."

Book design copyright © 2013 by Tate Publishing, LLC. All rights reserved.
Cover design by Rodrigo Adolfo
Interior design by Mary Jean Archival

Published in the United States of America

ISBN: 978-1-62563-275-3
1. Medical / Surgery / Transplant
2. Medical / Education & Training
13.02.12

Dedication

To Link Thompson, my incredibly generous donor who taught me that sometimes there is simply just no adequate way to say thank you.

To the simply extraordinary staff at the Mayo Clinic, Rochester, Minnesota, Kidney and Pancreas Transplant Center, who give life daily to those in their care.

To Bill and Helen Mills whom I first met when they were seemingly marooned on an endless waiting list and hope was ebbing away. Their successful living transplant a year later was my first experience coming alongside others in a situation similar to my own. It suggested to me that perhaps I had a gift for teaching and guiding patients and families during their consideration of kidney transplantation.

May a rich and abundant life be given to those who have certainly given both to me.

Contents

Foreword

Dear Reader,

Like half of us whose kidneys have failed, I first found out in the ER. And like most other stunned and scared patients, I knew almost nothing about kidneys, what makes them fail, how to get a new one, or what I was going to do next.

What we quickly learn about kidney failure is what victory looks like—a speedy and successful transplant. And what you learn from coaches like Woody Hayes is this: it's the game plan that determines success.

The game plan that Dr. Mark Wedel offers on these pages tells the transplant patient what move to make, when to make it, obstacles to anticipate, and ways to overcome them. This is up to date information sent in from up in the booth by a former player turned coach. Going into the biggest struggle you've ever been in with the outcome the most significant in your life, you want a view of the whole field. You need coaching, strategy, teamwork, and preparation. A good coach gives you the teaching, the strategy, the game plan, and the belief that inspires so that you too will join the thousands of kidney transplant patients who have made it into the end zone and scored. My friend and fellow transplant recipient, Mark, does that coaching here.

—Run Hard,
John Brockington
Green Bay Packers running back 1971–1977
NFL Rookie of the Year 1971
3 Time NFL Pro Bowler 1971-1973
Member of Woody Hayes' 1968 Ohio State
University National Championship team
Kidney transplant recipient 2001

Chapter 1

Why Write This Book?

Initially Overwhelming but Ultimately Life-Transforming

Kidney transplantation is an initially overwhelming—but ultimately life-transforming—event. It often descends upon us at a time in life when we least expect it. It comes when we aren't feeling well. It comes with implications that will impact every aspect of our lives, our health, our relationships, our emotions, our finances, and our future. It also comes with an obligation. The obligation is this: it is absolutely essential we get ourselves focused and educated for the colossal task at hand. We cannot even begin to prepare our hearts and minds for our transplant event without adequate education—good education and soon. Therein lies the problem. Educating oneself on all the issues related to kidney transplantation is a daunting task. Who will do the teaching? Where do the patient and family find the best information? From whom do patients and families seek counsel? Where are the reliable sources of information? What questions and topics require understanding? It is a daunting task indeed, if not just simply overwhelming.

The Need for Information Starts Early in the Journey

As personal testimony, I am a critical care physician whose career once involved caring for kidney transplant patients. My wife is a critical care nurse whose patients often included kidney transplant patients as well. Yet when it came our own personal turn to be on the receiving end of a kidney transplant, we were absolutely and completely lost. At that moment, it finally hit us: if we as health care professionals working right in the heart of the kidney transplant process were awash with confusion when our turn came, we could just imagine the plight of the average layperson trying to navigate the same challenges. This book is designed to help those patients and their loved ones who are considering kidney transplant. This book's purpose is to provide the necessary initial education so that they too can find a place in the rock of factual information to place their first anchor. It is only appropriate that those of us who have lived kidney transplant on both sides of the scalpel labor to fill that initial education void.

Comprehensive Education Materials for the Early Journey Can Be Hard to Find

Why is it so difficult to access good materials for self-education? Why is it so hard to get started? The reasons are several.

Transplant Centers

First, there are more than 250 kidney transplant centers in the United States. Extremely busy, dedicated, and highly talented individuals staff these centers. Their educational focus, however, is of necessity on the patients already entrusted to their care. In a perfect world, the transplant staffs would like to extend to you their total care and expertise. Unfortunately, there are only twenty-four hours in their days too. Virtually all transplant centers have their own education programs. These education programs actually range from quite good to simply excellent. They will be available once you have enrolled at your chosen transplant center. But choosing the transplant center that's specifically the best fit for you is not without its challenges. It is essential you be informed and educated well before that choice in order that you can play a role in your destiny. You will be teaming up with some of the finest doctors and nurses in the world at the transplant center you finally choose. You want to be a formidable and participating member of that team while on your journey. That simply means it is crucial we start the education right now.

To reiterate, some of the most important and fundamental transplant questions require answers before you ever first enroll at a specific site. For example, where is the best transplant center for your unique situation? Which transplant centers have the best outcomes? Which centers do the most transplants? If you are considering living donor transplantation, what transplant centers maximize your exposure to the largest number of potential donors? Which national registry, if any, is most ideal for you? If you anticipate being placed on the waiting list for a deceased-donor transplant, at how many centers do you plan to register on the waiting list? These are all questions that require your consideration *prior* to enrolling at a specific transplant center. In the chapters that follow, we will work through the logic process together. The time to start our education is now. Given the importance of what is at stake, let's get started.

The Internet

At this point you just might ask: why not simply use the Internet? In fact, my bet is that you've already tried it. After all, the Internet is an extraordinarily abundant source of information. Unfortunately—and I also bet I'm telling you what you've already learned on your own—the simple truth is that too much information can be as paralyzing as too little information. Google the search term *kidney failure* and you will get 12,600,000 hits in just 0.27 seconds. *Renal failure* will result in a harvest of 14,700,000 hits in under a half of a second. Even the search term *kidney transplant* returns more than 300,000 hits in an instant. No human being has the time to review 300,000 information sources, especially not those of us preparing for decisions that are becoming more imminent by the month. Not only is the sheer abundance of information overwhelming, but there is also an additional problem. The Internet has no editorial review board, no quality control officer, and no truth monitor. That leaves readers at our own peril as to whether information is truthful or which information has instead been generated by someone's vivid imagination or underlying agenda. Just because you read it on the Internet does not make it true. The risk of misleading information on the Internet is substantial.

The Extraordinary Progress in Kidney Transplantation

While all that may sound daunting on its face, the flip side of the coin is this: now is an absolutely wonderful time to be thinking about kidney transplantation. In fact, I submit to you that there has never been as fine an era as the present to be considering kidney transplant. I say this because three extraordinary medical accomplishments have all come together to create an unprecedented opportunity for kidney donors and their recipients.

Understanding the Long-Term Effects of Living Kidney Donation

The three notable areas of major medical advancement in kidney transplantation are the following: first, the natural history of living donors has been better defined. In simpler terms, that means large numbers of kidney donors have now been observed and studied throughout their entire lifetime in an effort to determine the long-term effects of living kidney donation. Specifically, this means physicians now have real data with which to counsel potential donors, real data to provide during the informed consent discussions. Physicians can now reassure patients that the life expectancy of living donors is the same, if not actually slightly longer than, non-donors. No longer are physician answers limited to best guesses or speculation based on only a year or two of observation following living donation. The lifetime health risks of kidney donation are now better described than ever before. We discuss these data, their implications, and their caveats in detail in the chapter on living donation (chapter 9).

Kidney Donation by Laparoscopy

The second of the three major medical advances is this: the surgical procedure for the living kidney donor is now virtually always performed laparoscopically. That means the extensive incisions of the older surgical procedures are now utilized only in rare and unusual situations. Today's laparoscopic technique uses two or three small incisions less than an inch long, along with a slightly larger midline incision to deliver the kidney. The result for kidney donors is earlier discharge from the hospital and more rapid recovery after donation. A decade ago it was anecdotally stated that kidney transplant surgery was harder for the kidney donor than for the kidney recipient. With laparoscopic surgical incisions for donors today, nothing could be further from the truth. Today the usual living donor is walking the afternoon of their surgery and leaves the hospital after a day or two of observation. We discuss this topic in detail in the chapter on living donation (chapter 9).

National Registries Can Expedite Matching Donors and Recipients

The third major advance is the extensive use of sophisticated computer matching registries that have vastly improved donor and recipient matching compatibility. These registries allow the pooling of large numbers of recipients and potential donors to improve each individual's odds of finding the best possible match. They simply use sophisticated computer software, developed specifically for this purpose, to provide the brainpower to do it. This remarkable phenomenon is revolutionizing living donor kidney transplantation. We discuss the mechanics of this major advance in transplantation in a subsequent chapter (chapters 7 and 8). Whether your transplant plans include living donation or deceased donation, the availability of this type of donor/recipient matching may prove to be a very significant factor in your determination of where you choose to receive your transplant. It is mandatory we understand these various matching programs well and consider them prior to our selection of a transplant center. Why? Because not every center participates in every registry, that's why.

You want to be sure that, if a matching registry is possibly in your future, you choose a site that participates in the registry most suited for your own personal situation.

TABLE 1. THE DECADE'S THREE MAJOR ADVANCES IN
KIDNEY TRANSPLANTATION

THREE MAJOR RECENT ADVANCES FOR PATIENTS CONSIDERING KIDNEY TRANSPLANTATION
Laparoscopic Surgical Approach to Kidney Donation
Defining the Long Term Natural History for Living Kidney Donors (risk)
Computerized Registries to Facilitate Donor: Recipient Matching

Moving Forward

As we journey through this book, we are going to walk together through a logical and generally chronological sequence of issues fundamental to your education about kidney transplantation. We will start with some immediate and important issues requiring thoughtful decisions even before we choose a specific transplant center. We will then make our way through information that will give us an important birds-eye view of the transplant process, preparing ourselves for our eventual choice of transplant centers. This exercise will aid us handsomely in preparing our initial battery of questions as we partner with our doctors, surgeons, and nurses at the transplant center where we will continue our journey. This journey will not be a sprint. Prepare for a marathon.

Why Write This Book? Take-Home Messages

- Kidney transplantation, while initially overwhelming, is ultimately life transforming.
- Education is critical to having a role in our ultimate outcome.
- Education will be a continuous process throughout our transplant journey.
- Education must start now because there are significant decisions to be made even before we are comfortably within the confines of our chosen transplant center.
- This is the best time in history to be considering kidney transplantation, thanks to three significant areas of recent progress
  - Definition of the long-term effects of kidney donation
  - Laparoscopic kidney donation
  - National registries to expedite the matching of donors & their recipients.

Chapter 2

You Are Not Alone.
Be Certain You Stay That Way

There is a time in the lives of all of us with kidney failure that we ask the "why me?" question. We feel as if we are the only person in whom kidney failure has ever occurred. Worse, many of us were just feeling a little out of sorts one day and then were diagnosed with kidney failure and informed of the need for dialysis the next. Surely we *must* be the only one, we think. But that perception is simply not the reality.

Kidney Disease Is Common Stuff

The reality is this: one in nine Americans has some degree of chronic kidney disease. Of concern, this number is increasing. At the end of 2009—the last year for which reliable numbers are available—more than 870,000 individuals were being treated for some form of kidney disease. Almost 400,000 patients were receiving dialysis in some 4,200 dialysis centers. Just under 200,000 people had functioning transplanted kidneys. You are *not* alone. You are *not* the only one with kidney failure.

Think about it for a minute, and you will realize there is some good news hidden in those statistics. The fact that a lot of individuals suffer from kidney failure means that the field of medicine devotes considerable time looking for ways to continuously improve available treatments. This is particularly true in the area of kidney transplantation. The kidney transplant world has seen phenomenal progress in the past half decade. Progress has ranged from the development of improved and less invasive surgical procedures for kidney donors to the improved understanding of any health effects related to kidney donation. The opportunities available to us from the science of kidney transplantation have never been greater. We are the fortunate ones.

At the same time, there are actually two sides to the coin of "being alone" with kidney disease. You just saw that a lot of Americans share the same illness we do. Now, as we turn our focus forward to the transplantation journey, "alone" takes on a different meeting. Just as we are not alone when it comes to having kidney disease, at the same time it is absolutely essential that we *not* attempt to make this journey alone either.

The Importance of Your Education and Your Support Team

You will have plenty of time later to meet other transplant patients, join transplant patient support groups, and participate in online support organizations. That will all come later. Now is the time when it is absolutely crucial that you establish the very foundation of your own personal support group. Discuss your situation and your planned journey with your spouse; your significant other; your parents; your children; your rabbi, priest, or pastor; your mentor; your primary confidante; your best friend; or whomever is appropriate. As you have these early discussions, make a decision as to which one or two or three of these individuals will be your greatest strength going forward. Tell them frankly and specifically that you want them to be at the core of your support. Include them in your journey right now as you begin your quest for information. Share what you've learned with them. Discuss with them what issues and questions you still need to pursue. Note well: this is not the time for "who will be my donor" discussions or simple informational updates that are often just "family press briefings." This is the time to put together your team, the best team you can find, the same team that will surround you as you ultimately complete your transplant journey. No one makes this journey alone. As the numbers above show, you are *not* alone. Now, as you begin preparing for your journey, it is absolutely essential that you stay that way.

You Are Not Alone. Be Certain You Stay That Way! Take-Home Messages

- You are not the only person to ever have kidney disease. You're in good company. One in nine Americans has kidney disease.
- Just as you are not alone in having kidney disease, do not try to begin your transplant journey alone either.
- Build the very core of your support team now.
- Involve them early and from the beginning in your education process.

Chapter 3

Why Would I Want to Choose the Kidney Transplantation Option over Dialysis?

Treatment Options for Kidney Failure

The universe of potential treatment options for kidney failure has just three major components: dialysis, kidney transplantation, and stem cell considerations. Stem cell science is exciting, frequently in the news, and proceeding at a prudent pace. However, while it is always risky to attempt to predict the pace of scientific progress, the widely held belief is that stem cell therapies will not be available as a treatment option in our lifetimes. As a result, we will dispense with further discussion of this exciting but still *Star Wars*-like treatment. That leaves us with dialysis and transplantation as our two basic treatment options.

Dialysis

Dialysis is the most common method for treating kidney failure. Four hundred thousand individual Americans receive life-saving dialysis therapy. Think of dialysis as existing in two varieties, hemodialysis and peritoneal dialysis. Furthermore, think of each of these two forms of dialysis as existing in two forms, in-center and at home. Traditionally, only about one in ten dialysis patients have received their dialysis at home. However, with recent advances in the technology and safety of dialysis equipment, there is a growing trend toward in-home treatment. This is good news because it offers the dialysis patient even more treatment options. An abundant patient literature already exists on dialysis therapies, and the subject of dialysis will not be further discussed here.

Kidney Transplantation

The other major option for the treatment of kidney failure is kidney transplantation. Just like with dialysis, kidney transplantation also exists in two different forms. Donor kidneys can come from living donors, or donor kidneys can come from deceased donors. Both methods have their distinct advantages and disadvantages. We discuss them in detail in chapter 5. For now, suffice it to say that approximately 175,000 Americans are living today with successfully transplanted, functioning kidneys. Additionally, another 16,000-plus transplants are done every year.

Freedom from the Activity Restrictions of Dialysis

Broadly speaking, there are significant advantages to kidney transplantation. First, transplantation frees us from the obligation to be present at the dialysis center a half dozen hours at least three times a week. Transportation time and logistics of travel back and forth to the dialysis center present an additional burden. Adding to the time burden is the issue of often feeling poorly as the result of chronic disease. It is not surprising that only about 10 percent of dialysis patients are able to work full time outside of their dialysis obligation. (Contrast that with the fact that more than half of transplanted patients return to full time employment.) Additionally, dialysis significantly impedes our ability to travel for work or for pleasure. While travel is certainly possible for dialysis patients when advance arrangements are made for interim dialysis in other remote dialysis centers, the logistics can be daunting. The freedom that transplantation patients regain, after being freed from dialysis, is simply extraordinary.

Freedom from the Dietary Restrictions of Dialysis

A second and much appreciated advantage of kidney transplantation is the ability post transplant to enjoy a normal diet and normal fluid intake. After years of severe fluid and diet restrictions, you will once again be consuming the foods that heretofore you have only dreamed of. Avocados, orange juice, a slice of pizza—all adventures that bring great joy to our human lives and all of which had earlier been high on our "do not touch" list—become permissible again. Happy days!

More Favorable Outcomes

The third major advantage of kidney transplantation over dialysis is found in the patient results. Groups of transplant patients, when compared to groups of dialysis patients, live longer. The ten-year survival for peritoneal dialysis is in the neighborhood of 9 percent. The ten-year survival for hemodialysis is approximately 10 percent. The ten-year survival for kidney transplantation exceeds 75 percent. These findings have now been verified in numerous different studies. Long-term patient outcomes are simply better with transplantation.

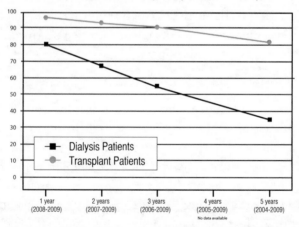

Graph 1. Graph showing improved patient survival from transplant compared to dialysis. At 85.5 percent, Note the 5-year survival rate for transplant patients (86%) is more than twice the 36% survival rate for dialysis patients (Data from National Kidney & Urologic Diseases Information Clearinghouse)

Lower Treatment Costs

The fourth advantage of kidney transplantation compared to dialysis is cost. The cost of kidney transplantation is significantly less than the cost of dialysis. For almost all Americans, Congress has determined that Medicare will be responsible for a very significant portion of our dialysis or transplantation costs. Still, while those costs may not come directly out of our own pockets, we as American citizens pay the taxes that fund Medicare. For that reason, there is at minimum a public policy reason to prefer kidney transplantation to dialysis. Indeed, the National Kidney Registry in a white-paper report estimates that the federal government could save ten billion dollars a year by placing emphasis on transplantation and a sophisticated national registry. (For further discussion of Medicare coverage of end stage kidney disease patients, see chapter 10.)

When Possible, Transplant Is Our Preferred Treatment Option

At the end of the day, kidney transplantation is clearly the superior form of treatment when compared to kidney dialysis. Yet not all of us are candidates for a kidney transplant. For those of us who do not qualify, should we despair? Of course not. Kidney dialysis is unquestionably a life-saving therapy. We should consider ourselves fortunate because dialysis is available to us. Like so many situations in life, we first consider our available options by ranking them in order of desirability. Then we shoot for the highest star attainable. The driver of the Buick needs not be embarrassed because they're not driving a Mercedes. The Olympic gymnast who proudly wears the silver medal does not despair her position on the reviewing stand. Similarly, for those of us whose kidney failure is being treated by dialysis, we rejoice because dialysis is certainly far more desirable than no available treatment option at all.

Before leaving this brief overview of available treatment options for those of us with kidney failure, we take a moment to discuss those people who have started on dialysis and then make the transition to a kidney transplant. Do people who have been treated with dialysis merit special considerations when considering transplant? Is there any interaction between the two therapies? In the most perfect world, the kidney transplant team would prefer that you and I have never been on dialysis. Indeed, in situations of living donation, your transplant team will try to time your kidney transplant to occur just as your kidney function has deteriorated to the point of requiring dialysis. This method of patient management is called "preemptive transplantation" and is the standard in most transplant centers today. The reason for the preemptive approach is found in the answer to the question: Is there any limit to how long I can be on dialysis before I get a kidney transplant? The simple answer is that there is no technical reason why transplant surgery cannot be performed on a patient who has been on dialysis for an extended period of time. There is, however, an abundant amount of literature to suggest the longer on dialysis, the greater and more negative the impact of dialysis on transplant outcome. There is no definitive agreement on how much dialysis will impact transplant results, but it is safe to say the best information suggests that dialysis longer than two to five years can adversely affect transplant results. Moral of the story: get going right now.

Why Would I Want to Choose the Kidney Transplantation Option over Dialysis? Take-Home Messages

- Our two main treatment options are dialysis or transplant.
- Dialysis is of two types: hemodialysis or peritoneal dialysis.
- Either form of dialysis can be done in a specialized center or at home.
- Two-thirds of people receiving these treatments today are on dialysis.
- One-third have functioning kidney transplants.
- Transplants can come from living donors or from deceased donors.
- Transplant is preferable to dialysis in terms of freedom of activity.
- Transplant is preferable to dialysis in terms of freedom of diet and fluids.

- Transplant is preferable to dialysis in terms of patient outcomes.
- Transplant is preferable to dialysis in terms of overall costs.

Chapter 4

Choosing a Kidney Transplant Center: What Considerations Should We Be Thinking About?

Education Is Key to Your Transplant Center Selection

Unfortunately, most of us do not choose our transplant center at all. Instead, we find ourselves enrolled at a particular center because our health insurance plan directed us there. Other times we just assume the center where our current medical team is working is the best center for us. While that might be true, it seems obvious that with more than 250 kidney transplant centers in the United States, there must certainly be differences between them. Sometimes those unique differences can result in a choice of transplant center that is better suited for our own unique situation. Given that our kidney transplant is likely the most significant medical-surgical event that will ever happen in our lives, it seems rather likely that we would want to play an active role in the choice of our transplant center. So where do we begin?

Finding Your Available Transplant Centers

First we are going to need to know the names and locations of all available kidney transplant centers. Fortunately, that list is easy to come by because the federal government keeps watch over all US kidney transplant centers. The information can be readily accessed on the website for the Scientific Registry of Transplant Recipients (SRTR) at http://www.srtr.org/csr/current/Centers/Default.aspx.

If you fill in your city and postal code, you will find the centers closest to you.

This information source is very reliable, run by independent scientists, and is free of commercial influence. It is a tremendously valuable website for kidney patients, our friends, and our families. In this book, we will refer to this website several times in our search for information that is specific to our own unique situations. For now, we will use this website to find all the available kidney transplant facilities in our particular geographic area. Another website that you may find helpful in your evaluation of potential transplant centers is www.konnectology.com. (Be aware, however, that this website charges a fee to cover operating expenses, hoping to avoid the potential bias that might be introduced by involving insurers, hospitals, or advertisers. You will find it considerably more user friendly than the government source, however.)

A third user-friendly resource can be found at http://www.kidneytransplantcenters.org. This site is provided by the National Kidney Registry, a nonprofit organization, and lists only those sites participating in the NKR registry but covers the institutions doing almost 75 percent of the kidney transplants that are done annually in the United States. Once we have determined our geographic options, we can address the unique questions we should be asking in order to decide among those choices.

Insurance May Affect Your Choice

Our first consideration will of necessity have to be our health insurance coverage. Mundane as this might sound, remember that our kidney transplant is, roughly speaking, a quarter of a million dollar investment. Only the rare individual could expect to complete the process without the benefit of health coverage, whether it is private or federal insurance. Many insurance plans direct their kidney transplant patients to specific centers. It makes no sense for any of us to be pursuing transplant sites outside of our insurance coverage, putting ourselves on the hook for $250,000 in the process. The message is: first learn all about your insurance coverage restrictions, if any. This information is generally available from two sources. First, a series of calls to your health insurance carrier will eventually bring clarity. Even better, most kidney transplant centers have dedicated health insurance coverage experts working specifically with transplant coverage and are frequently housed directly in the kidney transplant division. These individuals, when available, can be invaluable.

Transplant Center Results

The second consideration of importance for each of us will be the specific transplant center's outcome results, especially as that center's results compare to other centers available to us.

Additional information from that particular center is also pasted in the ten pages above Table B9 in the aforementioned SRTR website. Indeed, these pages are a veritable treasure trove of information about the transplant center you are studying. Patient survival rates one year after transplant are posted there. It is suggested that for our initial screen, the one-year survival rates are likely sufficient. Remember that when comparing one-year survival rates among different transplant centers, a 1 or 2 percent difference may not be "statistically significant," meaning simply that the complexities of statistics render very small differences meaningless. However, when our decision-making comes down to the final rounds, finding someone with an affinity for mathematics is a worthwhile exercise to aid in the digestion of the individual transplant center reports. Finally, the Konnectology website can also be of value here if you're willing to utilize a resource with an enrollment fee.

Transplant Center Level of Activity

A third important consideration will be the number of patients transplanted at any particular transplant center. As a general rule, one might infer that the greater the volume of transplants performed, the more polished and effective are the care systems in place in that facility. Practice makes perfect in many areas of life. The team that transplants frequently is likely to have better results than the team that doesn't transplant frequently, at least in general. Again, the number of patients transplanted annually is readily available from the SRTR website. While the volume of transplants done can be a reassuring figure, it does not necessarily mean that the busiest center is always the best center for the particularly unique among us. Is the Chevrolet from a mass-producing and robotized assembly line really a better car than the less common, partially handcrafted Lamborghini? Obviously volume of transplants done is just one consideration.

Transplant Center Waiting List Time

A fourth consideration of critical importance, especially for those of us anticipating a kidney from a deceased donor, is time on the waiting list. Almost one hundred thousand of us are currently waiting for kidneys. Worse, waiting list times are growing longer and longer. Importantly, know that waiting list times vary by institution, differing between central city and more rural institutions, with additional variation geographically. If we are waiting for a deceased kidney donor, it is absolutely essential that we be well informed about the average waiting time in our chosen institution. For those anticipating deceased-donor transplants, this may well be the most important consideration in our choice of regions in which to be transplanted. Information on how to obtain valid data on each center's waiting list time will be found in chapter 6.

Convenience

Fifth, of course, is the issue of convenience. Transplant evaluation is a very thorough and extensive process. Post transplant patient management, especially during the first month after transplant, is also a very intensive process. The result is an abundance of to and fro commuting and, if you are far away from home, a lot of nights away from home. If we have the choice of equivalent facilities but one is across town and the other one just down the street, convenience will favor the latter. When our choices don't include equivalent facilities, however, the balance becomes more difficult. We only hope to go through this incredible transplant experience once in our lives. If the cost of getting it right is limited to just the inconvenience of a few extra hours in traffic and a hotel bed, the choice is an easy one to make for most of us.

Being Listed at More Than One Center

Before closing out this discussion on our choice of transplant center, one critically important point still needs to be made. This point is aimed directly at those of us anticipating that we will be taking our place on the kidney waiting list for a deceased-donor kidney. Once we are approved, time on the waiting list will be our greatest obstacle. So, hear this: it is permissible to be listed on the waiting list at more than one site (provided they are in different Organ Procurement zones—a distinction to be explained later) at the same time. What does that mean for those of us waiting for a kidney? It means precisely this: when you've done your homework selecting your site for kidney transplantation, *select two sites*. This allows you the opportunity to choose one site with a very short waiting list but perhaps less personally convenient, along with a site with a longer waiting list but more convenient to your home and family. This is lawful and accepted behavior. A story that received much attention in the popular press was the story of Steve Jobs, CEO of Apple and the recipient of a liver transplant. Jobs was fortunate to have spent a relatively short time on the waiting list. Closer scrutiny of Jobs's strategy shows Jobs enrolled on the waiting list at a transplant facility with one of the nation's shortest waiting list times. Jobs was rewarded for his diligence by a waiting time that was significantly shorter than the waiting time at the transplant center in Jobs's local community.

The take-home message is clear: if at all possible and you are anticipating taking your place on the waiting list for a deceased kidney donor, you should be listed at more than one site. As always, check your coverage with your insurance carrier. Some, but not all, of your transplant evaluation studies will have to be repeated at the second site, and you do not want to incur non-covered expenses for those studies. Remember that most transplant centers will require you be available on site within a specific time, for example, six hours after being called. If a prospective recipient is unable to meet the time requirement, they will likely be passed over and miss their opportunity. Finally, as is the case with all transplant issues that occupy your mind, do not be anything but frank and forthcoming when discussing your motivation and site-selection strategy with your doctors and nurses.

Choosing a Kidney Transplant Center: What Considerations Should We Be Thinking About? Take-Home Messages

- Education is key to selecting the best transplant center for each of us.
- Just as we are unique individuals with unique situations, transplant centers are also unique.
- Making the best match between the transplant center and the patient is key.

- Among things to be considered in choosing the best transplant center for our needs are
  - Insurance coverage
  - Transplant results
  - Transplant volume
  - Expected waiting list time
  - Convenience

- Especially if you are considering a deceased-donor kidney, energetically investigate the idea of being listed at more than one transplant center

Chapter 5

Living Donation or After-Life Donation: What Are the Differences?

Earlier we noted that there are two major types of kidney transplantation: deceased donation (also known as cadaveric donation) and living donation. There are major differences between these two types of kidney transplantation in terms of preparation and outcome. It is important we understand these two options fully. First, however, we look at the history of kidney transplantation in America, and then we will compare and contrast the two types of donation.

The first successful human kidney transplantation was performed at Boston's Peter Bent Brigham Hospital in 1954. This first kidney transplant was a living kidney donation between identical twin brothers, Richard and Ronald Herrick, both of whom were in their early twenties.

The field of tissue and organ compatibility was just developing. The fact that these two pioneering patients were identical twins reduced some of the issues related to tissue compatibility. Still, this first ever whole organ transplant was the medical/surgical equivalent of landing a man on the moon. Richard Herrick lived eight years with his newly transplanted kidney. His donor brother Ronald died recently from complications of heart surgery at age seventy-nine. Chief transplant surgeon Joseph Murray received the Nobel Prize for his work. The important message from this story is the reassuring message that kidney transplantation has been going on for well over fifty years now. A lot has been learned. Tremendous strides continue to be made. That's good news for those of us who are going to need it!

Six years after the first pioneering living kidney transplantation in identical twins, the first successful deceased-donor kidney transplant was successfully carried out. This time the patient was treated with immunosuppressive drugs because the recipient was not related to his deceased donor. The successful procedure demonstrated that kidneys could also be successfully donated after life, providing even more hope for patients in kidney failure.

So now we have seen that there are two major forms of kidney transplantation, living donor and deceased donor. Next we will define these two forms of kidney transplantation more precisely, discuss their advantages and disadvantages, and then rank them in terms of their desirability.

Deceased-donor Kidneys

A deceased-donor kidney is one that is donated from an individual who has generously consented to gift their organ(s) after their death in order that others might live. The definition of the standard deceased donor (also known as Standard Criteria Donors or SCD) is a donor who has been declared brain dead by an independent neurologist and who, because of a catastrophic event, has zero chance of recovery. Recently, because of the inadequate number of available organs to meet the growing need for transplantable kidneys, several other categories of potential donors have been described. These are donors who by the most stringent criteria may have been considered less than ideal but are still likely to be able to make a significant contribution to others. These have included

- Expanded Criteria Donors (ECD), donors over fifty years of age who have some of the medical diagnoses associated with aging such as high blood pressure;
- Cardiac Death Donors (DCD or death after cardiac death) or donors who died of heart disease before a diagnosis of brain death could be established; and even
- High-Risk Social Behavior Donors, donors who at some point in their life practiced high-risk behavior for sexually transmitted diseases, drug usage, or were imprisoned but currently show no signs of active infection.

These non-standard donors all have donor kidneys that are perfectly reasonable organs for transplantation yet carry success rates that are perhaps 5-10 percent less than standard criteria donors. Not every center performs transplants on every variant of deceased donor. The result is that you need to explore with your chosen transplant center the types of donors they might make available to you.

Here is the important message for those of us anticipating being placed on the kidney waiting list: we *must* understand the various categories of donors and the potential risks of transplantation from each category. While this assignment is not an immediate one at this moment, it is imperative that once listed we must make our decision *immediately* as to which categories of donors we are willing to accept. Next we need to share it with our transplant team. *No individual is ever forced to accept a kidney about which they are not fully informed*. No transplant team will ever make the decision for you. *You* are responsible for that decision. The moment that an organ is available for you is *not* the time to be considering these issues for the first time. That moment is too filled with other emotions and the necessary details of preparation for surgery. It is not a time when one can reasonably expect to make good and rational decisions regarding complex issues not previously considered. This is your responsibility. Execute it as carefully and diligently as you execute any of the important tasks that deal with the well-being of you and your family.

Living Donor Kidneys

Living donor transplantation, on the other hand, is the procedure where the donor kidney is removed from an otherwise healthy person and surgically placed into the recipient with kidney failure. The donor is generally a relative, a spouse, or a friend, but can even be a total, and extraordinarily altruistic, stranger. Most often the procedures are carried out simultaneously in adjacent operating rooms. While the recipient is being prepared for receipt of a new kidney from the surgical team in one operating room, the donor kidney is being surgically removed by another transplant team just yards away in a separate operating room. Less often, the kidney is removed in one operating room and then flown to the operating room in the city where the recipient lives.

Advantages of Living Donor Kidneys

Which is the preferable procedure: living donation or a deceased-donor kidney transplant? There is no question. While both procedures are life saving, a living donor is preferred for the following reasons:

Living Donor Kidneys Outcome

First and foremost, the success rate of living donor kidneys is higher. This fact has been demonstrated time and time again in large scientific studies. Results from living donation have shown that the life of the living kidney is approximately twice that of the deceased-donor kidney. It has been further shown the poorest-matched (in terms of HLA matching) living kidney is still better than the best-matched deceased-donor kidney. Abundant data now confirms the main take-home point here: a living donor kidney is preferable to a deceased-donor kidney.

Living Donor Recipients Avoid the Waiting List

Other less important benefits also come from living donor kidneys: first, having a living donor means the transplant recipient will avoid the waiting list for a deceased-donor kidney. Whenever possible, the uncertainty of the waiting list and the growing amount of time spent on that waiting list are best avoided. Living donation avoids the list (note, however, that even candidates with expected living donors are nevertheless placed on the waiting list as a contingency, the future being no more predictable in kidney transplantation than anywhere else in life).

Living Donor Kidneys Function Sooner

Second, the living donor's transplanted kidney begins to function almost immediately, often within minutes of surgically reestablishing the kidney's blood supply. Deceased-donor kidneys can take days or weeks to begin functioning. This avoids any consideration of having to undergo dialysis post transplant while waiting for the transplanted deceased-donor kidney to begin functioning.

Living Donor Transplants Can Be Scheduled Electively

Third, living donation can be planned and electively scheduled. This minimizes the chaos and frenzy related to the uncertainty and unpredictability inherent in deceased-donor kidneys. A scheduled surgical procedure is of benefit to everyone. Clearly in the hierarchy of desirable outcomes, the opportunity to have a living donor is clearly at the very top of the list.

Living Donation or After-Life Donation: What Are the Differences? Take-Home Messages

- Kidney transplantation has been going on for more than fifty years now.
- The kidney recipient has two donor options: a deceased donor or a living donor kidney donation.
- Both forms of kidney donation can be life saving.
- Living kidney donation is preferable to deceased donation in terms of
  - Outcome
  - No waiting list time
  - Virtually immediate kidney function
  - Elective preparation and scheduling

Chapter 6

The Waiting List: What Is It All About, and What Does It Mean for Me?

The waiting list actually applies to all of us, whether we anticipate a living donor or a deceased donor. Virtually all experts in the field recommend initially listing all transplant candidates, even those subjects anticipating a living donor. The simple reason is that even living donation is not a reality until after the transplant is actually finished. In the meantime, it behooves all of us to start accruing time on the waiting list. The result is that the "waiting list" information found in this chapter is appropriate for all of us, regardless of the type of kidney donor we are anticipating. But first, some history:

The Government's Role in Maintaining the Waiting List

All us of are at least somewhat aware of our government's role in regulating tissue donation. In fact, one might correctly consider organ transplantation to be the most regulated portion of an already heavily regulated US health care system. The involvement of the government in end-stage kidney disease first had its origin in legislation written by Senator Al Gore and signed by President Richard Nixon (see chapter 10). This legislation was initially directed at patients with end-stage kidney disease but, as remarkable medical and surgical advances in kidney transplantation were taking place, a system for organized and equitable distribution of organs became necessary. In 1984, Congress passed the National Organ Transplant Act (NOTA). NOTA mandated the scientific registry for transplant patients (SRTR, www.srtr.com) and established the formation of the Organ Procurement and Transplant Network (OPTN). The purpose of the OPTN is to insure uniform quality in transplant centers, ensure fair and equitable distribution of donor organs, and to protect the deceased donor's family members during this sensitive and vulnerable period. The OPTN is the only organ procurement organization in the United States and is administered by the United Network of Organ Sharing (UNOS). An abundant amount of literature exists describing the goals, ethical issues, and mechanics of operation of this federal system. For our purposes here, it should be sufficient to know that the program has multiple internal reviews, built-in cross-check mechanisms to ensure fair and equitable organ distribution, and is run with regular input and advice from medical professionals from both inside and outside the field of transplantation.

As a general rule, as soon as a candidate is accepted for transplantation, the transplant center immediately places the candidate onto this "waiting list." UNOS will confirm your place on the waiting list with a letter. Be certain you receive yours.

Supply and Demand Inequality Results in the Waiting List

The most important implication of the waiting list is found in the mathematics of the "waiting list" equation. The sobering numbers are these: there are currently more than 90,000 patients on the waiting list for a kidney. Every day eighteen people on the waiting list die, still waiting for a kidney. In 2011 alone, more than 4,700 patients died while still waiting. Because the amount of kidney disease in our population increases each year, the waiting list grows larger each year. In fact, the waiting list has increased by 25 percent in just the past seven years. Waiting times similarly grow and now can easily exceed an average of five or more years, especially in large urban areas. If we consider the reported median dialysis patient survival times and compare that to patients' median time on a waiting list, we quickly recognize with alarm that in some areas, particularly large urban areas and in large states like California and Texas, the median waiting time can exceed the median survival on dialysis. The result: eighteen of us die every day, still waiting. All of this just serves to remind us of the tremendous organ shortage and the resultant unmet medical need. There simply are not enough donor organs to meet the need. Of course, none of this is meant to decry deceased-donor donation. Successful deceased-donor kidney transplantations are done every day in the United States. These efforts result in thousands of saved lives. Recently the number of living donors surpassed the number of deceased kidney donors, yet because each deceased donor enables *two* recipients to be transplanted, the total number of deceased-donor transplants still exceeds the total number of living-donor transplants.

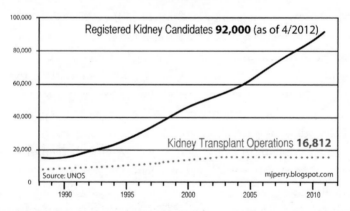

UNOS data showing the growing discrepancy between the growth of the kidney transplant waiting list and the number of kidney transplants performed annually, from mjperry.blogspot.com

Learning the Waiting List Time for any
Specific Transplant Center

Chapter 4 advised us that when choosing our transplant center, the center's waiting list time could be a very important consideration. Once again, the Scientific Registry of Transplant Patients (SRTR), www.srtr.org, is an extraordinary resource. Follow this pathway below. If you are not successful on your first effort, be patient and try it again. Here is the map:

1. Go to the SRTR website, www.srtr.org.
2. In the upper right-hand corner of the screen, under PSR Quick Links; click on Transplant Program Reports.
3. Next, click on the Kidney box.
4. Now scroll up and down to find the transplant center you are interested in and on the far right of the center's listing, click on New Format.
5. Scroll down about ten pages to Table B9.
6. On the far left of the screen, find the line that says 50th percentile (median time to transplant). The number immediately to its right under Center is the average waiting time in months for patients on that center's waiting list.

Of course the problem here is that this data is information necessarily based on a center's *past* performance. How do we predict the future? Well, we can't. But Garet Hil, who arguably has the largest observational experience in the world of kidney matching, outlines a formula for approximating expected waiting times in the future. In his book, *Finding a Kidney and Getting the Most Out of Your Transplant* (Xlibris Publishing, 2011), Hil suggests we look at the number of patients on a center's waiting list, divide it by the number of deceased-donor transplants done the previous year, and then divide that number by two (to correct for the attrition of patients from the waiting list) to get a number representing the prospective waiting time in years for patients currently being listed. For example: if a center has one hundred patients on the waiting list, transplanted ten deceased-donor kidneys the past year, the Hil calculation suggests a waiting time of five years (one hundred divided by ten is ten, and ten divided by two is five, suggesting a five-year waiting list).

Finally, there are also websites specifically designed to help individuals find the transplant centers with the shortest waiting time closest to their homes www.konnectology. com. This is likely the easiest site to use but does require an enrollment fee.

Collecting information on transplant center waiting times for patients with your unique situation is *not* a trivial pursuit. Unquestionably the best way to deal with the waiting list is to avoid it. The best way to avoid it is by pursuing living-donor transplantation if at all possible.

The result is that planning for and securing living donation should ideally be our highest priority.

In passing, we will note that currently one of the most important factors in determining one's place on the waiting list is time already spent on the list. Children, along with individuals who have already been living donors, receive special consideration. Medical urgency, compatibility, size match, and proximity of the donor to the recipient are additional determinants. Kidneys are always made available to local patients first. The country is divided into eleven geographic regions, each managed by a single organ procurement organization. The geographic regions are further divided into a total of fifty-eight donation districts. Available kidneys are always offered first in the donation district where they occur. When no suitable match can be found in that district, only then are they offered to patients in other nearby geographic regions. Wealth, fame, notoriety, race, or ethnic background carry no value and do not affect one's place on the waiting list.

You may have once thought that waiting for a deceased kidney donor would be a far easier task than ever discussing your need for a kidney with family or friends. Now that you've been introduced to the complexities of the waiting list, however, you may wish to reconsider the relative difficulties of the two tasks. The next chapter will introduce you to the issue of talking with prospective donors.

Dr. Mark K. Wedel, MD, FACP

The Debate Over the Ideal System
for Kidney Allocation

Of course, there will always be an ongoing debate over the most perfect system for determining one's place on the waiting list. The current system emphasizes that the waiting list system must at all times be equitable and fair to all. An alternative school of thought melds in some degree of utilitarianism; for example, the youngest donor kidneys go to the youngest recipients because of the longer life expectancies of both the kidney and the recipient. In this paradigm, the fundamental emphasis on organ distribution goes from "waiting time" to "expected survival." One calculation suggests that transition to this new modified system would add ten thousand life years of survival each year it is in use. At this point in time, however, while the debate is ongoing, Americans traditionally seem to have preferred the current system that emphasizes fairness and equitability to efficiency and utilitarianism.

The issues involved, however, are worth the consideration of all of us, especially those of us who are directly or indirectly involved. While the entire ethical debate regarding living donation is beyond the scope of this writing, these are nevertheless profound issues to be considered by all of us. Starting on the one hand with the acknowledgment that kidney-donor surgery is the only surgical procedure in all of medicine where the patient operated on receives no certain medical benefit, and moving to the other hand with the thought that perhaps the world's richest country might be obligated to develop a more efficient solution to this growing kidney supply and demand issue, you might see things a little differently. As you ponder the medical need of the patients on the waiting list and the current allocation of an inadequate number of transplantable organs, do yourself a favor and consider the passionate and persuasive writing of Virginia Postrel, author and altruistic kidney donor. Ms. Postrel's credo is manifest in her choice of title "...With Functioning Kidneys for All." Surely, Postrel argues, we can find enough kidney donors for those who need transplants. But "doing so will require creativity, boldness, and a sense of urgency—and experimenting with controversial ideas like donor chains and financial incentives." The sense of urgency is shared by all of us. I believe it imperative we embrace the "creativity and boldness" of her call to arms.

http://www.theatlantic.com/magazine/archive/2009/07/with-functioning-kidneys-for-all/307587/

One current example that might qualify as "creative and bold" might be found in the proposed revision of the current system of allocating kidneys, a system, as mentioned earlier, based primarily on length of the patient's waiting time. One recent computer simulation has suggested that a revised allocation system could add ten thousand life-years annually to kidney failure patients per year, simply by use of the same policy that's already utilized in heart, liver, and lung transplants. This proposal suggests taking the 20 percent "best" deceased-donor kidneys and matching them first with the 20 percent "best" potential recipients, a match that is heavily influenced by age. In such a system, the youngest of available kidneys would not likely be going to a recipient with an otherwise shortened life expectancy, for example, from advanced age. Conversely, a donor kidney with shortened life expectancy would not be going to the youngest person on the waiting list. The remaining 80 percent of kidneys would be distributed just as we currently do it, meaning 80 percent of us would likely see no change in the system. As mentioned, this is the way available hearts, livers, and lungs have always been shared. One objection is that such a system might represent subtle age discrimination. Another questions whether we can really trust the predictive formulas that attempt to define the "best" donor kidneys and the "best" recipients (http://www.ustransplant.org/pdf/Wolfe_LYFT_ROTSOT_07.pdf).

The Importance of Being an Advocate

I promised you early on in this book that kidney transplantation would be a life-transforming event for you. Start girding yourself now with the information you'll need *after* transplant to further the health and lives of others who have exactly the same needs we all have had. Once transplanted, you never depart the transplant family. Kidney transplantation will be a life-transforming event for you. You can never repay those who will do so much for you but you can try, so start now.

The Waiting List: What Is It All About and What Does It Mean for Me? Take-Home Messages

- Supply-and-demand inequality results in a waiting list for kidneys
- The waiting list is not kind to those who are waiting
- Waiting time varies from center to center, region to region
- It is vital to know the waiting times at the centers you are considering
- Finding a living donor eliminates our need for a waiting list
- Creativity and boldness are required if we are to find a better solution than a waiting list
- Who more than those of us with the need to answer that call?

Chapter 7

How Will I Ever Find a Donor?

Remember that at the very outset of this book I told you that now is an unprecedented and ideal moment in time to be considering kidney transplantation. Three major medical advances have all converged in recent years to result in this marvelous opportunity. To refresh, the first was the introduction of laparoscopic kidney removal from living donors. The second major advance is the improved understanding of the long-term natural history of living kidney donors. Here is the third one: highly sophisticated computer software that allows for a far more ideal system of matching donors and recipients. We will describe this advancement shortly under the heading of "paired donation."

Our approach to this topic will involve two primary areas of emphasis. The first item of importance will deal with the tactical aspects of discussing your need for a kidney donor with your family and friends. We will then move to the topic of national, computer-matched registries or so-called "paired donation." The latter phenomenon is making a rapid and substantial contribution toward facilitating matching and decreasing matching times, all by providing kidney patients with wider access to potential living donors.

Your search for a donor will begin with your small circle of family and friends but then often widens into a larger and more populous world of potential donors in the national registries. This is why we will start with a discussion of your initial conversation with family members and friends, and then move toward a discussion of the national registries and their potential value in your search.

Communicating Your Need for a Kidney Donor with Others

Over the years I bet you have asked the people closest to you to help you out with all sorts of things—a ride home, a sandwich, a glass of ice water, a golf tee, even a few dollars. But a kidney? No way. A kidney seems to most of us to be way beyond the pale.

But here's the incredible secret. You are going to be surprised to learn how many people there are in this world and in your own circle of family and friends who are filled with an unbelievable generosity and goodness of spirit. Their generosity is so profound that they will consider your plight without you even asking them. I bet you are living among heroes and didn't even know it. All they need from you is to know about your need. You won't need to beg. You won't need to sell. You simply need to communicate. Without knowing your situation, your friends can never seriously consider their ability to meet your need. That means your task is to inform them. Informing is still a complex task, but it is less formidable than "asking" for a kidney. It is key to remember this because it is so much easier to get a task done successfully when we are focused on the right task, not the wrong one. Remember, this is all about informing people. It is not asking them.

Another excellent learning resource comes from Harvey Mysel, a Chicago businessman and kidney recipient. Mysel has developed a website at www.LKDN.org, a site that is an excellent resource for learning the approach to discussing our need for a kidney when we talk with others. Mysel advocates the "elevator speech," meaning a brief response to the question, "Hello, how are you?" that could be given in the time it takes the elevator to leave the first floor and arrive at the top floor. In essence, it enables the patient to welcome the questioner's greeting and then acknowledge that there is a current struggle with kidney disease going on and that it is going to require a kidney transplant. That is the essence of an effective initial conversation. The seed of need has been planted. If the seed germinates at all, additional information can be given in a subsequent conversation. See also *http:// www.livenow.info/GetLiving/IntimacyRelationships/Telling OthersAboutYourChronicKidneyDisease.aspx* for additional information as well as the unique idea of having business cards made to help tell your story.

Transplant center coordinators are also often invaluable resources for these subsequent conversations. Indeed, UNOS directs that a potential donor be given their own personal advocate within the transplant center, thus providing an excellent opportunity for continued education as well as the protection of the well-being of the potential donor.

Indeed, in the current era of social media, even resources such as Facebook, Craigslist, Twitter, and YouTube have resulted in people responding to an individual's succinctly stated needs. A recent survey of Facebook posts seeking kidney donation found ninety-one ads from patients ranging in age from two to ninety-one years, 12 percent of whom were transplanted and another 30 percent of whom reported potential donors had stepped forward to be tested. The review was appropriately critical of the fact that only 5 percent of the posts mentioned risks, and only 11 percent mentioned the possibility of associated costs for the donor. Moral of the story: If you choose to go the social media route, it works, but in the course of your social media conversations, it would be well to make mention of the issues of side effects and potential costs (chapter 9) as well.

Finally, rest assured that everyone recognizes this is a difficult task to learn. Know that your chosen transplant center will also provide individuals and resources to assist you in this process, often providing educational materials and volunteering to sit with families and potential donors in conversation about living donation.

Just who might be appropriate for initial conversation is fairly straightforward; family members, especially siblings, come immediately to mind. Close friends, spouse, close coworkers, confidantes, and mentors all come to mind. Prior to the widespread use of "paired donation" and national registries, tissue compatibility was a paramount issue in considering potential donors. We will discuss the mechanics of compatibility testing of donors in chapter 9. We will touch on the topic of compatibility testing in this chapter for recipients as well as again in the chapter for donors (chapter 9). It involves both of you, so we will do it twice, each time in small bites, so that you both understand. Before doing that, however, it is necessary to understand the revolution occurring with paired donation and national kidney donor registries.

The Initial Step in Screening for a Potential Donor

Recall that the first living kidney transplant in history was done between identical twins. Since most of us do not have the (good?) fortune of having an identical twin, tissue compatibility between donor and recipient becomes highly relevant. The mechanics of tissue compatibility can be considered in three steps. The very first step is blood typing. Donors and recipients must have compatible blood types. A table of blood type compatibilities is shown here:

ABO BLOOD TYPE COMPATIBILITIES

You	Donor is O	Donor is A	Donor is B	Donor is AB
O	Yes	No	No	No
A	Yes	Yes	No	No
B	Yes	No	Yes	No
AB	Yes	Yes	Yes	Yes

You can see that an O *donor* is compatible with another O, an A, a B, or an AB recipient. At the same time, see that an O *recipient* can *only* receive from an O donor. This is the reason O blood types are sometimes referred to as "universal donors" (ignoring Rh factor considerations for the time being). On the other hand, note that an AB *recipient* can receive from any type of donor, whereas an AB *donor* may only donate to an AB recipient. This results in the description of AB blood types as "universal recipients" (again, ignoring Rh factor considerations). The biology behind blood-type matching and incompatibility is fairly simple, and if you are interested pursue the topic at *www. khanacademy.org*. For the time being, however, and for the sake of simplicity, just use the table. Note that Rh positivity or negativity is irrelevant to our transplant compatibility conversation. That means that an O blood type is considered as an O, whether it's O positive or O negative. For the sake of thoroughness note also that in rare circumstances blood-type compatibility is not an absolute necessity. These circumstances, however, are quite rare, and the complexity of those cases is beyond the scope of this manual.

So that you might better appreciate the uniqueness of your own personal blood type, the relative percentage of people with various blood types is as follows.

BLOOD TYPE FREQUENCIES

BLOOD TYPE	DONOR IS B
O	45%
A	40%
B	11%
AB	4%

Remember that we initially established that there are three steps in the tissue compatibility testing, the initial step being blood typing. The next two steps are human leukocyte antigen (HLA) testing and, finally, cross matching. These latter two steps are deferred to chapter 9. Here we want to stay on the topic of blood-type compatibility to drive home the fundamental concepts behind "paired donation."

Paired Donation, Local, and National Registries

Let us imagine for a moment that Pair #1's husband needs a kidney transplant and is blood type A. Further imagine that Pair #1's wife wishes to be her husband's donor, but she is blood type B. The ABO compatibility table shows you that this transplant would be incompatible and could not be undertaken. Blood type B cannot donate to blood type A.

Now imagine a second pair, Pair #2, where the husband needs a kidney transplant and is blood type B. Further imagine that Pair #2's wife wishes to be her husband's donor, but she is blood type A. The table again shows you that this transplant would be incompatible and could not be undertaken either. Blood type A cannot donate to blood type B.

Left to their own devices, neither of these husbands in need of a kidney transplant could be transplanted. But if the two couples were to be "paired" with each other, Wife #1 with her B blood type is a perfectly compatible donor for Husband #2 and his B blood type. At the same time, Wife #2 with her A blood type would be a perfectly compatible donor for Husband #1 and his A blood type. The result is that if both these transplants are performed at the same time—Wife #1 donating to Husband #2 and Wife #2 donating to Husband #1—two patients who previously had no compatible donors now each have compatible donors and can be successfully transplanted. This is the fundamental principle behind paired donation—that is, the pool of recipients and donors is broadened enabling a greater mathematical probability that compatible living donor transplants can take place.

It then follows that if more matches can be made by considering two couples at a time, would there not be reason to believe that the more individuals there are in the pool, the more likely it would be to find matches in an expanded pool? The answer is yes, this is indeed the case. When the pool gets larger, the mathematics behind determining the best matches becomes increasingly complex, ultimately requiring sophisticated computer software to do the calculations. Nevertheless, the outcome is intuitively obvious—more matches, lessened waiting time, and greater efficiency dealing with extremely difficult matches. To date, the longest chain of "paired donation" consisted of sixty patients, thirty donors and thirty recipients. In the next chapter we will review some data to demonstrate that what had been theoretically obvious is now reality. The advent of computer software sufficient to perform these incredibly complex mathematical calculations is a major advance in donor-recipient matching and is truly one of the great breakthroughs in kidney transplantation in this decade.

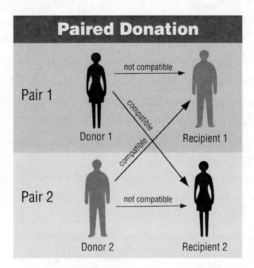

The fundamental lesson from this chapter is that computerized matching systems have greatly facilitated matching. Entry into living donor programs generally requires that each of us have our own living donor identified. If every volunteer donor were a perfect match for his or her intended recipient, we never would have needed computerized matching. That is just not always the case, however. Sometimes the donor is incompatible or perhaps just poorly compatible. In that case, while we know the donor is perfectly compatible with someone else somewhere else, the question becomes how to identify that ideal recipient. Even more important, the question is how to link that recipient's potential donor to our own need and, in exchange, enable someone else to have access to a donor ideal for our own situation. But how do we find those connections? How do we make that match? There are nonprofit programs that will do this for us and, in fact, are doing it for people every day. Each of us as needs to consider the following: are we going to rely simply on our own resources for finding a donor, or are we going to expand our access to the pool of potential living donors by seeking potential assistance from a registry? Key to making this decision is realizing that there are multiple programs being used by multiple transplant institutions. They come in all sizes from large to very small, from those with a track record to those just having started, and with different amounts of published data on both short- and long-term success. Not every matching program is available in every transplant center. Some programs (for example, the Mayo Clinic) have their own intramural paired donation program, offering the advantage of common protocols and practices and finances. For this reason, investigate the registries (chapter 8) and investigate what registries the centers you are considering are currently using. Start the process of making your decision *now*! First, do I want to consider using a matching program if I cannot find a compatible donor? Second, which matching program would I hope to access? Finally, does my preferred transplant center offer access to that particular program, and, if not, which one(s) do they use or have they created their own?

How Will I Ever Find a Donor? Take-Home Messages

- Learning to inform your family and friends of your current battle is an important skill.
- Abundant resources exist to aid you in learning this skill.
- It's about informing, not asking.
- Determining your ABO compatibility with potential donors is a first step in the matching process.
- Paired Donation allows incompatible donors to save another's life and, in return, have their donor save yours.

Chapter 8

Paired Donations and National Registries: Should I Be Personally Involved?

My answer to you is a categorical yes. The rhetorical question back to you is, why would you *not* be involved? Here are the reasons you want to be involved:

At Best, a Registry Provides a Kidney; at Worst, It Provides a Back-Up Plan

First, even though you may believe you have already found your healthy donor, until you are actually transplanted you have no guarantee that your proposed donor will actually be your donor. What if your donor becomes ill? What if your donor's circumstances change? What if they change their mind? As you are aware, things can change. The old adage "hope for the best and prepare for the worst" is certainly applicable here.

The Possibility of a Better Donor: Recipient Match

Second, it may be that an exchange program can provide you with a donor who is an even better histocompatibility match for you than your current prospective donor. If your prospective donor is willing to participate in such an exchange, consider paired donation as a potential mechanism for bettering your match. The data that supports the rationale for this particular use of paired donation is only now beginning to develop. However, the early data does trend in the direction of support for this approach. Consider *all* your options. A few percentage points of increased survival every time you improve your donor's HLA matching with your own will result. How important are those few extra percentage points of survival to you? My bet is that they *are* important to you. Just remember that time is of the essence. Considering improving your match is fine only when it does not delay your transplant. If a delay in time to transplant is involved, discard the idea immediately.

The Larger the Pool of Prospective Donors, the Greater the Likelihood of a Match

Third, people who are going to be difficult to match are more likely to be matched if multiple prospective donors, rather than just a single or several individuals, are being considered. People who are going to be difficult to match include those with a prior transplant, those with prior blood transfusions, or those with high levels of circulating antibodies (otherwise known as high panel reactive antibodies—or PRA scores). Remember that even pregnancy, in view of the cross-circulation between mother's blood and the placental circulation, can sometimes result in antibodies that render histocompatibility matching problematic.

Large Registries May Result in Shorter Waiting Times

Fourth, data accumulated to date by the National Kidney Registry shows a shorter waiting time for patients enrolled in their registry compared to those outside the registry, currently about six months in the registry and longer outside it.

The take-home lesson is clearly this: investigate the various national registries. Ask the important questions: (a) How many transplants have you matched? (b) How many and which hospitals are you affiliated with? (c) How often does your registry's computer do matching runs? Finally, (d) what are the one and three year results of those patients you have matched? Know well the transplant centers you are considering, and then make your decision. See the Additional Resources chapter at the end of this book for a partial listing of registries.

Paired Donations and National Registries: Should I Be Personally Involved? Take-Home Messages

- Kidney registries can provide a larger pool of potential donors than otherwise available to us on our own.
- Registries *may* be able to provide us with a better match than we currently have.
- Registries *may* be of particular value for those of us who are hard to match.
- Registries *may* enable an earlier match than otherwise possible.
- It is very important to know the characteristics of the various registries, their history, their number of successful matches, and which of them participate with the transplant center you are contemplating.

Chapter 9

What Does the Potential Living Donor Need to Know?

Donors are heroes. There is no other way to put it. Donors save lives. They give life to kidney patients whose life is ebbing away. Donors give hope to the families and loved ones of those suffering from kidney failure. Donors are the cornerstones of kidney transplantation. Donors are simply beyond incredible!

In this chapter, we will initially begin with a discussion of the requirements for being a donor. A closer consideration of the topic of "tissue matching" will follow. Finally, we will go into a very careful discussion of "informed consent," that is, a full and detailed description of all the risks potentially inherent in kidney donation: short term, long term, and otherwise.

As we said at the outset, donors have truly magnanimous hearts. In my own personal situation as a kidney recipient, I still find it impossible to find appropriate words to describe the size of the heart that characterizes my donor. We salute all of you, even if you're only just beginning to give this undertaking some thought. We all think we know the benefits of donating a kidney—that is, we save another person's life. But consider this: recently an altruistic donor, in his words, "...wanted to give a stranger a second shot at life." When his paired donation chain finally ended, a total of sixty individuals were involved! Can any of us even fathom the magnitude of generosity that saves thirty lives and pours out joy upon sixty families?

Qualifying to Be a Living Donor

Transplant centers require that donors, first of all, be in impeccable health. Mild blood pressure elevation or mild blood sugar elevations can often be reasons for exclusion. Simply being overweight, for example, can be a reason for disqualification. Surprisingly, age is not necessarily a hindrance. While younger kidneys are always more durable than older kidneys, older kidneys are certainly better than no donor kidneys at all. The team at Johns Hopkins studied more than twenty donors over the age of seventy. They concluded, if you are over seventy and in good health, you are not too old to donate a kidney.

No carefully controlled multicenter studies have ever been conducted to determine precisely the best medical tests to use for determining donor eligibility. As a result, significant variability still remains among transplant centers when examining the specific criteria used to define an acceptable candidate. This is probably most often seen in the area of blood pressure elevation. For example, some centers will not allow any blood pressure elevation; an equal number will allow blood pressure elevations that are controlled by a single medication, while a minority will allow blood pressure elevations that are controlled by two medications. This basic message is this: the acceptance criteria for being a donor are very high. The only way you can know for sure is to find out. The first step is usually a simple screening interview, either over the telephone or online, answering basic questions about your health history.

After passing their screening interview, donors are then evaluated by those tests normally recommended and appropriate for the donor's age and gender. For example, in addition to routine history, a complete physical exam and routine blood tests, if your age and gender recommends you have mammograms, mammograms will be done (if that requirement hasn't already been recently satisfied). If your age suggests colonoscopy is an appropriate screening procedure, colonoscopy will be required. At the same time, if you are younger than the age at which routine colonoscopy is normally recommended, colonoscopy will not necessarily be routinely required.

Beyond that evaluation, certain additional tests are required to aid in the transplant process. For example, tests will be done to assure you and that you actually have two kidneys (one in 750 of us is born with only a single kidney). The surgeons need to know your kidneys' size, how many blood vessels supply your kidneys, and where they are.

In addition to your physical evaluation, donors are also routinely evaluated from a psychological perspective. Transplant teams need to know for certain that an individual's motive is a positive one—that is, they are not motivated by money, notoriety, or some other unrealistic expectation. Because there is no 100 percent guarantee that every kidney transplant will be successful, the team requires assurance that a prospective donor is aware of this fact and knows that while an immediate transplant failure is quite rare, it can still happen. Both the transplant team and the prospective donor must be prepared to deal with such an unusual outcome. Remember that UNOS requires that all prospective donors have their own donor advocate. The prospective donor's evaluation is carried out entirely independent of the recipient's evaluation. Information is not shared between donor and recipient during the evaluation process in order that the prospective donor may be entirely free of external influences as they contemplate their decision.

Finally, your team will begin to inquire to as your current level of informed consent. We will discuss informed consent in detail in a few pages, but for our purposes here, understand that the evaluation team is preparing you for a complete understanding of the journey you are about to undertake.

When you consider the profound benefits of kidney donation and the complexity of fully understanding the potential risks involved, you will understand that the donor evaluation process is of necessity carried out with great care and diligence. There is no hurry-up to this evaluation. Personally, I believe some delay is actually built in to the donor evaluation process on purpose. This is for the protection of donors. Six months from volunteering to donation is probably a pretty typical figure. Knowing what you need to know and thinking about it carefully and thoroughly takes time. You should never be rushed.

The more correct terminology for our "matching" discussion is probably "donor tissue type characterization." This is because the donor's tissue characterization happens first, and only then is a decision made as to whether or not there is compatibility between that donor and the intended recipient. As we have seen above, however, every donor is always a perfect match for someone, somewhere. The immediate question is whether the donor's intended recipient is a match or whether a paired donation will be required in order to transplant that intended recipient.

Matching Donors and Recipients

As we implied earlier, tissue characterization (so-called "matching") happens in three steps. First, blood type is determined. Table 1 showed us the compatibilities of our various blood types. This is your first step in your look at compatibility with a potential donor. If your blood types are compatible, your "matching" process proceeds to the second step. Even when a donor believes they know their blood type, blood type is always reconfirmed by the transplant center. Most often, after passing the screening interview by telephone or online application, the transplant site will either invite the prospective donor to the center for blood tests to determine the individual's blood type, or, alternatively, the center will send the potential donor a mailing kit so their blood can be drawn locally and then shipped to the transplant site for final determination.

The second step in tissue characterization of the donor is called HLA determination. HLA stands for human leukocyte antigen, a modestly complicated immunologic phenomenon that, fortunately, no donor or recipient needs to fully understand. The simplified version of HLA testing goes like this: each of us has six HLA antigens. The more donor antigens that match the recipient's antigens, the better is the match. For example, six out of six antigen matches occur in identical twins. Most siblings are (statistically) most likely to have three of six matching antigens. But here is the important thing to remember: while it is true that the greater the number of HLA matches, the better the long-term survival results, the differences between one or two antigens is not substantially different from matching four or five antigens. The point is that HLA matching needs to be kept in perspective. The more HLA matches there are, the better, but "better" is a relatively small percentage. Remember, a 6/6 match from a deceased-donor kidney is still not as good—in terms of graft survival—as a 0/6 match from a living donor.

MATCHES	0	1	2	3	4	5	6
10 yr SURVIVAL	54%	56%	59%	57%	59%	62%	73%

Living Donor Graft Survival Rate at Ten Years and
Number of HLA Antigens That Matched

The final step in tissue typing and cross matching is a laboratory test in which the donor's blood is mixed directly with the recipient's blood to be sure that antibodies from the recipient do not attack the tissue of the donor. This test measures the tissue compatibility of the specific donor and specific recipient and absolutely must be passed in order to proceed with transplant.

So for the moment we will assume that either compatibility testing is underway or that it has been successfully completed. What else does the prospective living donor need to know? We will divide this discussion into short-term risks, long-term risks, and miscellaneous risks. Remember that UNOS requires that your transplant center appoint an "independent donor advocate" to advocate for your needs, rights, and interests in the process. This is to protect you as a potential donor from any real or perceived coercion. It also guarantees that you as a potential donor consider your own situation independent of the pressures involving the potential recipient. Your advocate will also be heavily involved in teaching you the necessary information to ensure your consent is informed.

To understand potential short-term risk, the prospective donor much consider two events related to your surgical procedure: first, general anesthesia and second, the surgical incisions.

Informed Consent and the Potential Risks of Living Donation

Speaking in broad terms, it can be stated that on the whole, living donation is safe with few perioperative deaths, complications, or long-term medical issues. Several truisms are commonly stated about the risks. For example, the risk of dying during kidney donation (0.03%, or 3 in 10,000) is equivalent to sky diving twice, or driving 20,000 miles, or driving 40 miles to work for a year. It is important, however, for us to go well beyond these generalities and look at the specifics.

General Anesthesia

Kidney donation surgery is carried out under general anesthesia. General anesthesia is administered under the supervision of an anesthesiologist. General anesthesia is a routine part of virtually every surgical procedure done every day in every hospital in every part of the world. However, it is *not* perfectly safe. General anesthesia does not come with a 100 percent guarantee. There are always risks, no matter how rare. This is a topic certainly worthy of quality discussion with your anesthesia team.

Surgical Incisions

Another aspect of kidney donation is the surgical incisions themselves. Remember that today the vast majority of kidney donations are carried out laparoscopically. We earlier described the laparoscopic method of kidney removal as one of the three major medical advances in kidney transplantation. Not every transplant center, however, is routinely doing laparoscopic removal. Be sure you are aware of the method your transplant center is using. Your postoperative course is significantly longer and more arduous if the older surgical approach is used. Of course, regardless of surgical method, all surgeries create incisions, and all incisions are at risk for postoperative infections. There are also several other less common complications that can occur. Again, they are worthy of quality discussion with your surgical team.

The usual kidney donor is admitted to the hospital the day of the planned procedure. When operated laparoscopically, the donor is usually ambulating with assistance by the end of the day. You will stay in hospital for observation to assure your vital signs are stable, you are taking fluids and foods by mouth satisfactorily, and that your incisional pain is satisfactorily controlled with oral analgesics. Most institutions prefer you stay a day and a half or two after surgery before you can be discharged. This is a very cautious and prudent approach, but you deserve it. You're the hero, and absolutely no one wants you exposed to any unnecessary risk.

Post-Operative Pain and Discomfort

Probably the biggest post-operative annoyance for kidney donors is "gas" in their abdomen after surgery. In order to have sufficient room to "see" laparoscopically inside the abdominal cavity, it is routine that during the laparoscopic procedure, carbon dioxide gas is delivered into the abdominal cavity. Carbon dioxide is the gas you breathe out when you exhale. It is the gas that puts the fizz in your soda. If you were to view your abdomen from the outside during surgery, your abdomen would look distended as if you had "a lot of gas." In reality, however, the gas is not inside of your stomach or your intestines but *outside* of your intestines but still *inside* the abdominal cavity. After the carbon dioxide gas has served its purpose of improving the surgeons' ability to see their operative field, it remains behind when the surgery is completed. Eventually it will be completely absorbed by the body. In the meanwhile, however, the body's process of absorbing that gas is rather slow, meaning it may well still be present five to seven days hence. The gas can annoy other organs in the abdomen and result in discomfort in the shoulders, back, or abdomen overall. In my experience, the most common post-operative complaint from donors results from this collection of gas and the discomfort it produces. Most donors refer to it not so much as pain but as annoying, a nuisance, or a need to burp or throw up. Expect it. It is likely the most annoying part of your whole journey.

Long-Term Side Effects of Living Kidney Donation

The question about the long-term safety of kidney donation is also relevant for donors. For many years, medicine simply *assumed* donating a kidney was not harmful in the long run. Most of that assumption came from physicians' anecdotal experiences with their kidney donors. The belief was further buttressed by the fact that 1 in 750 of us are born with only a single kidney and generally don't appear to have any long-term effects from it. However, no one really *knew* because there was no significant large data set about donors that carefully studied donors' long-term outcomes. Fortunately, larger data sets now exist, and significant portions of the question have now been answered. The larger data set was gathered by the University of Minnesota and suggested the following: for donors, no long-term increase in the risk of cardiovascular or cerebrovascular disease, no increase in kidney disease, and no shortening of life expectancy. (In fact, in the large Minnesota study, donors appeared to outlive non-donors by approximately two years, but that's an observation suited for multiple statistical arguments and a good one for you to discuss with your statistician friends; http://www.nejm.org/doi/full/10.1056/NEJMoa0804883.)

It is my belief that the determination of long-term health outcomes for donors is one of the three great developments in kidney transplantation of our era. The reason is because we as physicians no longer have to offer "best guesses" of reassurance but instead can now look at a significant scientific database and draw these conclusions. There is one important caveat about this data, however: the Minnesota data largely reflects the Minnesota population where Scandinavians and northern Europeans are heavily represented. *The data, therefore, may not necessarily be directly applicable to other ethnic groups, black Americans, Hispanic Americans, Native Americans, for example.* That data remains to be gathered analyzed. How can you help? Insist on being followed up long-term by your transplant center. "Long term" means for the rest of your life. Even if you move to another location, lab tests can easily be performed in one city and analyzed in another. Our profession did not do a very good job of long-term follow-up of donors in the early years of kidney transplantation. In fact, despite the fact that our living donors are the very cornerstone of kidney transplantation, it was not until 2000, almost fifty years after the first living donor kidney transplant, that UNOS required centers to report at least one year of follow-up data on donors to OPTN. As professionals, we ought to be embarrassed by that. We are, and we are all committed to doing it better in the future. Your insistence provides both support and encouragement to get it right.

Returning to Work after Kidney Donation

A final post-operative issue is your return-to-work date. Again, this is highly variable and depends on your age, your pre-operative physical fitness, your occupational requirements (desk work or manual labor, for example), and the rapidity with which your intra-abdominal carbon dioxide is absorbed. Your surgical center will give you their recommendations. They will always be conservative. You will likely surpass all their predictions. But hey, what is the hurry? You've just done a very heroic thing. Now you deserve everyone's best care in order to guarantee you the very best possible outcome. Remember that many states have now enacted legislation that requires employers to allow employees to take time off for organ donation. Some of these statutes forbid employers from subtracting this time from accrued vacation and even guarantee that your job is waiting for you upon your return. California's law, for example, requires companies with more than fifteen employees to grant up to thirty days of paid, work-protected leave for kidney donation. Even better, some institutions (e.g., Mayo Clinic) actually encourage organ donation by granting additional time off to their employees who donate. If you are working, get in front of your Human Resources representative and get your options defined for you.

Dr. Mark K. Wedel, MD, FACP

Potential Social Implications of Living Kidney Donation

Finally, in addition to the possibility of short-term and long-term complications from donation surgery, there are potential social implications for you to consider. First, there are instances of perfectly healthy donors who have been denied medical insurance after their successful donation. This is not routine, but there are instances where insurance companies have declared kidney donors as having a "pre-existing condition." Given the information about long-term donor outcomes that we've just discussed, this blanket insurance decision is certainly nonsensical. Unfortunately, it has been the occasional reality. Other insurance companies reasonably require the successful completion of blood tests that verify the health of the individual who has donated. Recently passed federal legislation suggests the concept of "pre-existing condition" may go away, but unfortunately that same legislation doesn't prohibit a significant increase in the premiums for these "pre-existing condition" people.

Consider also what might happen if an unexpected condition is found during the donor's screening evaluation. It could potentially result in a "pre-existing condition" and uninsurability for the donor. These are obviously worst possible scenarios for donors, but every donor is entitled to be aware of the possibility. So just beware. These are mostly minor problems but are certainly not minor for the individuals to whom they happen.

Medical Costs for the Living Kidney Donor

The second potential social implication for donors is the potential for incidental medical costs. The routine situation is that the donor's medical expenses are covered by the recipient's health insurance policy, even when the latter is Medicare.

However, events such as travel to and from the transplant center, lodging during the donor evaluation process, and lost wages from missed work are not covered. Sometimes recipients will have the means and the largesse to cover these costs for the donor, but technically, the donor is responsible. Just be aware.

Finally, a handful of personal stories from donors can be found in the bibliography at the end of this book. They are worth a few minutes of your time.

You as a donor are about to embark on what is potentially the most noble and generous life-saving activity of your lifetime. You are the very cornerstone of kidney transplantation. Remember that at the same time, however, from the other side of the coin your kidney donation surgery can also be viewed sternly but legitimately as the only surgical operation that provides absolutely no physical benefit to the person undergoing the surgery. The result is that risk: benefit considerations and donor safety are a serious obligation for all of us, not just those of us who are hoping to donate to save a life, but also for the physicians, surgeons, and nurses charged with taking care of us. Get yourself educated!

What Does the Potential Living Donor Need to Know? Take-Home Messages

- Donors are heroes, period.
- Donors must be in very good health.
- The health evaluation for prospective donors is excellent and thorough.
- Every transplant center provides prospective donors with his or her own personal advocate for their donor journey.
- The compatibility between recipient and prospective donor continues from the original ABO blood type determination, now to HLA antigen testing and finally to the search for recipient antibodies hostile to the prospective donor's kidney.
- Informed consent is critically important for every prospective donor.
- Informed consent covers many elements, including short-term, intermediate-term, and long-term risks as well as potential social and financial implications.

Chapter 10

The Unique and Complex World of Health Insurance Coverage for Kidney Transplant Recipients and Living Kidney Donors: Do I Really Have to Get Involved?

Health insurance coverage is, by its very nature, always complex and always in a state of flux. No simple summary could ever be written. Nothing written today about coverage is necessarily still correct tomorrow. But before dealing with the hard parts, we should take a look at the positive side of health insurance coverage. Kidney failure is the one illness in the United States that comes closest to having universal coverage for US citizens. Thanks to Medicare, currently 92-93 percent of Americans are eligible for coverage for kidney failure, dialysis, and/or transplantation. Just how did such a fortunate circumstance for kidney patients come about?

Dr. Mark K. Wedel, MD, FACP

The History of Medicare Insurance for Virtually All Kidney Failure Patients

On October 30, 1972, President Richard Nixon signed the Social Security Amendments of 1972, one provision of which automatically extended Medicare coverage to persons with kidney failure. That amendment became law in July of 1973. It meant that *any* individual with kidney failure, regardless of age, was automatically granted Medicare coverage *provided that they were otherwise qualified for Medicare (defined by ten years working and contributing to the program, or having a spouse or parent that met those same eligibility criteria).* Political pundits have suggested that the general expectation of the Capitol Hill politicians in those years was that some form of national health insurance would very shortly become political reality. Therefore, they figured, our population of kidney disease patients was a great pilot population in which to test the waters of universal care. When you realize that today we are talking about treatment options of dialysis with a price tag of $75,000 per year, or transplant at a cost of $250,000 for just the transplant *per se*, or even the necessary post transplant immunosuppressive drugs at a cost of $1200 per month, what a blessing. It's a rare individual indeed who could stand to shoulder these costs personally. The situation is made still worse by the fact that most of us come into dialysis or transplantation as chronically ill individuals, often unable to work and thereby no longer covered by workplace health insurance. So for all of us with kidney failure, what a blessing!

Of course, as with all insurance, there are always complexities. For example, if you have group health insurance from your employer, your employer will remain your primary insurer for the first thirty months after transplant while Medicare serves as your secondary insurer. Following the thirty months, Medicare becomes your primary insurer and your group health plan, if still in effect, becomes your secondary insurer. This transition period is euphemistically called *coordination of benefits*, likely a term only a politician could coin for the legislation that mandated it. Complexities like *coordination of benefits* are best dealt with on an individual basis in consultation with your insurance company or your employment's human resources department. While complex, the coverage is always a blessing. Most transplant centers have insurance coordinators and experts to guide you through the maze. These individuals can be real godsends.

The Extraordinary Cost to Medicare for our Medical Coverage

We know that every blessing has an opposite side and that relatively universal Medicare coverage for kidney disease patients is no exception. The major issue here is the cost of the program to Medicare. The original budget for this program when it originated in 1972 was $135 million.

Today that same budget is $20 billion. Of course, the number of patients in the United States with kidney failure in 1972—at the time of the original legislation—was only 10,000. You know that today's population of kidney disease patients—either on dialysis or with functioning transplants—now numbers 600,000. Imagine the havoc on your own household budget if a necessary commodity like gasoline were to increase 15,000 percent. Do you think you'd still be driving?

The point here is simply this: we kidney patients all need to recognize our good fortune when it comes to Medicare coverage. At the same time, we need to be sensitive to the pressures on those charged with administering and paying for our benefits. The clashing pressures are, of necessity, going to result in a litany of changes in the system. Expect them. Understand them, and remember to be thankful for what we already have.

Of course, the Medicare system is not perfect. No health insurance system is. Two salient issues to be aware of are these: first, as currently written, Medicare coverage for the necessary post transplant immunosuppressive drugs ends thirty-six months after transplant *unless* the recipient has reached traditional Medicare beneficiary age. The result is that younger patients who have not yet reached the traditional Medicare beneficiary age are left with a medication cost in the neighborhood of $12,000 to $15,000 per year. Commonly this is a financial burden they cannot meet. Often private health insurance has not been available to them, the result being the financially driven cessation of necessary medications and the ultimate loss of the transplanted kidney. Back they go to dialysis ($75,000 per year) and up goes the cost of their care to a much higher level than the cost of their medications ($15,000 per year) would have been. Cost benefit analyses have suggested that government action to eliminate the three-year restriction for these individuals would save Medicare $200 million per year. Legislation to correct this shortsightedness is currently in committee somewhere on Capitol Hill. If you're talking to your elected representative, take advantage of the opportunity to make a plea for both financial and medical common sense. The loss of transplanted kidneys in young individuals because of this three-year limit is a very real problem. Frankly, it's a tragedy.

The second issue worthy of your consideration is this: remember that the cost to the government of hemodialysis for a year averages $75,000. The cost to the government for peritoneal dialysis averages $50,000. The annual cost to the government for a kidney transplant, on the other hand, averages $18,000 per year. You and I established earlier that kidney transplantation is clearly our preferred treatment in terms of longevity and quality of life. Since even we non-accountants can easily see the cost savings of a national policy that emphasizes kidney transplantation as the preferred therapy for kidney failure, it is easy to see the need for thoughtful and creative ways to affect this emphasis. Remembering that transplantation is currently limited by the number of available kidneys and remembering that the 1972 legislation prohibited the sale or purchase of organs in the United States, start your own creative thinking about incentives to living donation like tax incentives, tuition credits, and other in-kind benefits. This debate is not new, is complicated, and is beyond the scope of this text. However, know that the original legislation by Senator Gore in 1972 was accompanied by writings that said the proscription of organ sales was a good starting place; the proscription may have to be revisited in the future. I suggest to you the future is here.

Earlier I told you the universe of health care coverage, rules and regulations, is constantly changing. That was an understatement. Yet constant change is not an excuse for failing to master this challenging topic as you prepare for transplantation. The most important reason I can think of is that some of these choices, for example, whether to pursue at-home dialysis versus in-center dialysis, will affect the starting dates of your Medicare coverage. Surely you wouldn't want to be making the decision re home versus in-center dialysis without knowing that one particular choice may initiate your insurance coverage as much as three months sooner than the other. Be informed.

Using the Experts to Help You Understand Health Insurance Coverage

So what to do? Fortunately, all major transplant centers have professionals whose sole duty is to understand coverage, coordinate benefits, and provide information to their center's kidney patients. Believe me, they can be some of your most valued friends. Get in front of them just as soon as you've made your choice of transplant center.

Second, certain insurance agents providing private insurance coverage often specialize in the coverage of kidney patients. Use your local kidney support group to search for individuals competent in this area. Visit them. Even Medicare will put choices in front of you, choices like "gap" insurance and Part D for medication coverage. Maximize the information at your fingertips. Many of the opportunities to make the best insurance coverage decisions have expiration dates. Hindsight is 20/20. Hindsight in the kidney transplant area equates with lost opportunity and often lost dollars. Frustration is guaranteed to occasionally infiltrate your efforts. Expect it. Resolve not to let it affect your efforts. Learning the insurance system is a battle in which you must prevail.

The Unique and Complex World of Health Insurance Coverage for Kidney Transplant Recipients and Living Kidney Donors: Do I Really Have to Get Involved?
Take-Home Messages

- Health insurance for kidney failure patients is complex and seemingly always in a state of flux.
- Most kidney disease patients requiring dialysis or transplant automatically are receive Medicare coverage, regardless of age.
- Medicare coverage for kidney patients is an extraordinary blessing for us as patients while placing a substantial financial pressure on the government's taxpayers.
- This financial pressure results in the constant change in the specifics of our insurance coverage and should be understood and expected.
- A basic mastery of the general rules of insurance coverage is essential as uninformed insurance decisions can be expensive to the patient and are often irreversible.
- Transplant center insurance experts, as well as local, private insurance agents can be tremendously helpful.

Chapter 11

What Will Post-Operative Immunosuppression and My Daily Pill Regimen Be Like?

Kidney transplant patients always require intra-operative and post-operative immunosuppression, in other words, a cocktail of drugs to keep the body from rejecting the newly transplanted kidney. There is variability in the drugs used by different transplant centers and for different patient needs. Much research is currently underway searching for even better immunosuppression regimens. For those reasons, this topic is best dealt with in detail when you are recovering from your transplant and a post-operative immunosuppressive program is being tailor-made specifically for you by your transplant team. Nevertheless, there are some generalities that are appropriate to mention here because it is absolutely key that you understand them thoroughly.

Post-Transplant Immunosuppression Drugs

First, your post-operative medical regimen will consist of multiple medications, likely more than you have ever taken in your life. Just your immunosuppression regimen alone will likely include three drugs (although a third of sites today are using steroid sparing regimens). You will have to keep your medications well organized. The timing of your medications is critical. You will have to keep *yourself* well organized. You will have to establish a regular routine. The reason is that it is critical that you maintain a steady blood level of your medications at all times. Wide fluctuations in the amount of drug in your bloodstream from hour to hour only increase your chances of side effects and diminish the drugs' effectiveness. Don't ever put your new kidney at risk! A smart phone with an alarm can be very helpful. So is a pill box. So is establishing a regular time every day that is religiously followed for medication taking. Our medications cannot help us if we do not take them or if we take them haphazardly. It is time to get religious about pill taking.

Blood tests that measure the amount of medication in your system are critical to the success of your transplant team's designer-made immunosuppression program for you. In fact, initially these blood levels may be determined on a daily basis until your team has determined the perfect dose for you. Of course, if you are haphazard in the timing of when you take your medications, these tests only generate false information and interfere with your team's efforts to design the best possible program for you. Get religious about pill taking, remember?

Medication Side Effects

Side effects, of course, occur with all medications, and your transplant team will discuss extensively with you the nature of potential side effects. There are two side effects, however, that are worth mentioning in general. The first is that immunosuppression, while good for maintaining the health of our transplanted kidneys, also slightly impairs our body's natural cancer surveillance defense system. As a result, cancers occur with approximately twice their normal frequency in those of us who are immunosuppressed compared to those who aren't. A large share of these cancers is skin cancer. The take-home message for kidney transplant patients is that we must become super vigilant about skin cancer, seeing our dermatologists regularly for screening, and becoming absolutely compulsive about regular and appropriate use of sunscreens.

The Dollar Costs of Immunosuppression

A second "side effect" is that of cost. The average immunosuppression program costs approximately $12-15,000 per year. Fortunately, for those with Medicare Part B coverage, this is a covered cost. The coverage lasts three years, at which time it continues if the kidney recipient would normally have qualified for Medicare but ends if the patient is still too young to be Medicare eligible. Legislation is currently being reviewed on Capitol Hill to reverse this significant oversight in the kidney transplant coverage system.

Orders, Not Suggestions

At the end of the day, understand this: you will likely be taking more medications than you ever have taken before. These medications are absolutely critical to your post-transplant success. Your transplant team's instructions to you are orders, not suggestions. You must develop the discipline to take these medications regularly and faithfully as instructed by your team. Finally, your team will carefully and repeatedly instruct you in potential medication-related side effects. This is all a routine part of successful kidney transplantation. All those who have gone before you have successfully navigated their way through it and continue to work and enjoy normal lives. Follow their lead.

What Will Post-Operative Immunosuppression and My Daily Pill Regimen Be Like? Take-Home Messages

- Post transplant, you will likely regularly be taking more medicines than you have ever taken in your life.
- Your medication program will be custom designed for you by your transplant team.
- These medications *must* be taken regularly and on time.

- Your transplant team's medication directions are orders, not suggestions.
- Potential side effects are myriad and will be discussed in detail with you by your transplant team once your individual program has been designed.
- Two things to be aware of re these medications: the data suggesting an increase in tumors and their substantial cost.

Chapter 12

Should I Be Considering My International Options for Transplant?

Should you consider having your kidney transplant done in a country other than the United States, perhaps to save some money, perhaps to have an easier time finding a donor? In a word, *no*. Although the World Health Organization estimates that a kidney is illegally traded every hour worldwide, there are several reasons this is a situation you absolutely want to avoid.

Illegal and Unethical Options Do Exist

First, you are correct in understanding that kidney donors and kidney transplant are available in other countries of the world. You can search out these sites on the Internet. You can read about kidneys available for purchase. You can find the contact numbers of individuals who claim they can facilitate your "transplant tourism."

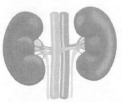

Why It Is Imperative We Avoid Them

Poor Oversight

First, we've mentioned earlier that kidney transplants are heavily regulated in the United States. One of the benefits of this regulation is that you are able to access legitimate and truthful data about a transplant center's patient volumes and their success rate. Because all of this data is scrutinized and juried by third-party experts, you can bet your life on its accuracy. On the other hand, when you search websites of non-US transplant centers, you will find claims as to patient volumes and results, but they are only claims. Third-party verification of what is claimed by these sites on the Internet is totally absent. Further, it does not exist. You are putting your life in the hands of someone who claims to be expert, but remember, all you get is a claim.

Managing Complications

Second, imagine that during your operative or post-operative course you develop complications. Do you know for a fact that your third-world center will be able to manage your complication? Will they be *willing* to manage your complication? What if your complication is a long-term complication, e.g., Hepatitis B or Hepatitis C resulting from inadequate infection control techniques? Where will you get treatment for this lifelong complication? Is it reasonable to expect the US healthcare system and your fellow US citizens to now shoulder the consequences and burden of your decision to be transplanted abroad?

Abusing the Less Fortunate

Third, how about the donor in a third-world country? Can you live with the idea that the donor may have been coerced? Can you really believe the donor's right to full informed consent was fulfilled? Can you be certain the donor will receive the appropriate lifelong follow-up care? News sources are replete with stories of organs from executed prisoners, government dissidents, the destitute and vulnerable, even a report of a youngster who traded a kidney for an iPad. The World Health Organization (WHO) reports that 40-50 percent of some Pakistani villagers have only one kidney, having given away the other one in return for compensation. But also according to WHO, more than half the money from this illegal organ trade goes to the middlemen who coerce these organs out of the poverty stricken. Are these stories all true? Who is to say for certain? But it is axiomatic that where there is smoke, there is fire. I am sure none of us wish to be party to any actions that would encourage such activities.

Avoid It at All Costs

Remember, our appropriate regulatory agencies, our appropriate safeguards, and our appropriate patient and donor advocates systems are entirely absent. You will never know for certain in advance what the real truth is. I hazard to say, even when completed, it is not likely you will know the whole story then either. Kidney donation must be a free will decision, period. Kidney recipients must have the best available treatment and follow-up, period. Neither of these requirements can be guaranteed in overseas and third-world transplant centers. Do *not* do it.

Should I Be Considering My International Options for Transplant? Take-Home Messages

- Illegal and unethical third-world options do exist.
- These programs can present a real danger not only to you and I as patients but also to the unfortunate people whom they exploit.
- The risks are real, the benefits uncertain.
- Don't do it.

Chapter 13

Finally, What Are Reasonable Expectations for My Outcome?

Of course, as is the case in every area of medicine, there are no guarantees. But first we can paint a broad-brush picture of what is generally true. When looking at large numbers of transplant patients over the past two decades, there has been remarkable progress in short-term survival. Results in one-, three-, and five-year graft and patient survival have steadily improved. That's the good news for all of us. As a rule of thumb, it is probably fair to figure that the average transplanted living donor kidney recipient can expect to receive an additional ten years of life. One-year survival rates are greater than 90 percent. A three-year survival rate of 93 percent was recently reported. Ten-year survival approaches 75 percent. These are extraordinary numbers representing extraordinary accomplishment by our transplant teams. But as we all know, these are only statistics, and statistics only apply to large populations. Each of us, on the other hand, is an individual, and there is only one number that applies to us—that is, the number reflecting our own outcome.

Statistics Apply to Populations but
Our Own Result Is Personal

Since each of us has only one outcome, I suggest we use the numbers above as a bookmark to give us a general idea of realistic expectations. Next we commit ourselves to becoming the exception. One of Dr. Thomas Starzl's original transplant patients clocks his fiftieth year post transplant later this year. That particular gentleman does not even require immunosuppression any longer. So with a potential range of outcomes from immediate rejection while still in the operating room to fifty years of post-transplant survival, I suggest we fix our crosshairs on the fifty years end of the spectrum.

After transplant, we all recognize that we have been given a second life. We celebrate that and live our lives remembering the gift we have received. Rejoice. Celebrate. Be thankful. Take your medications regularly and on time. Follow the standard rules that maximize good health. Follow a prudent diet, exercise, rest well, and be healthy in spirit. In partnership with your transplant team, manage your blood pressure, your cholesterol, and your blood sugar. You are a perishable item. Live accordingly.

You and your family are about to experience one of the most extraordinary experiences of a human lifetime. Get yourself fully prepared, and embrace the opportunity fully. You will never regret it. I am not telling you it is going to be easy, but I am telling you this: it is going to be worth it.

Finally, What Are Reasonable Expectations for My Outcome? Take-Home Messages

- Long-term results from kidney transplantation are, if nothing else, miracles.
- Acquaint yourself with these reasonable expectations.
- At the same time, remember these numbers apply to large populations of people, not to individuals.
- Each of us is an individual, empowered to maximize our own benefits.
- Embrace the challenge.
- No one said this will be easy, but everyone says this will be worth it!

Additional Resources
and References

Why Write This Book?

This is the story of the first successful kidney transplant between identical twins in 1954, an inspiring and courageous story that serves as framework for this entire discussion.

*http://news.harvard.edu/gazette/story/2011/09/a-transplant
-makes-history/*

Several excellent navigators covering many topics of relevance to the area of kidney transplantation:

*http://www.kidneylink.org/KidneyTransplantBasics.aspx
www.konnectology.com
www.transplantcafe.com*

You Are Not Alone. Be Certain You Stay That Way!

National Kidney and Urologic Diseases Information Clearinghouse: government sponsored through the National Institute for Health (NIH), one of the very best sources for numerical information about kidney disease in the United States: *http://kidney.niddk.nih.gov/KUDiseases/pubs/kustats/index.aspx*

Why Would I Want to Choose the Kidney Transplantation Option Over Dialysis?

National Kidney Foundation: the national parent organization for kidney disease and the founder of the 'End the Waiting List' program. A multitude of resources for the kidney patient are available at this very extensive website: *www.kidney.org*

American Association of Kidney Patients: a national nonprofit funded by kidney pts for kidney pts, goal is education and to improve health and well-being of CKD patients: *www.aakp.org*

A Nobel laureate warns against untested "rogue" stem cell therapies: *http://www.reuters.com/article/2012/10/09/us-nobel-medicine-yamanaka-idUSBRE8980E920121009*

Kidneylink: a comprehensive resource on kidney transplantation written and reviewed by medical professionals: *www.Kidneylink.org*

Choosing a Kidney Transplant Center: What Considerations Should We Be Thinking About?

Scientific Registry of Transplant Recipients: provides a profile on each US transplant center, the number of patients transplanted each year, as well as their patient results: *www.srtr.com*

Konnectology: a fee for service resource that provides extensive information on transplant centers and their results and specialty areas: *www.konnectology.com*

An Internet blog for transplant related issues that contain another précis about choosing a transplant site: *http://transplantheadquarters.blogspot.com/2007/03/how-to-look-up-transplant-center.html*

Organ Procurement and Transplant Network: essentially the data arm for UNOS; it maintains the only national waiting list and contains very comprehensive data on transplant waiting lists and outcomes: *http://optn.transplant.hrsa.gov*

Living Donation or After-Life Donation: What Are the Differences?

United Network for Organ Sharing: a private nonprofit that manages the USA's organ transplant system under contract with the federal government. The NOTA (National Organ Transplant Act) of 1984 called for a private nonprofit to run the Organ Placement and Transplant Network (OPTN). Has held the federal contract since 1986: *www.UNOS.org*

The Waiting List: What Is It All About, and What Does It Mean for Me?

Waiting times at individual transplant centers can be viewed at *http://transplantheadquarters.blogspot.com/2007/03/how-to-look-up-transplant-center.html*

An excellent summary of the transplant process and paired donation registries, as well as Hil's proposed formula for prospectively calculating waiting list times, can be found in *Finding a Kidney And Getting the Most Out of Your Transplant, Garet Hil, author, www.xlibris.com,* 2011 (order at Orders@Xlibris.com)

A thoughtful article by author and kidney donor Virginia Postrel: "…With Functioning Kidneys for All." The author Virginia Postrel argues, "Surely we can find enough kidney donors for those who need transplants but doing so will require creativity, boldness and a sense of urgency…"

http://www.kidneyregistry.org/pages/p25/TheAtlantic_VirginiaPostel_709.php

The debate over the best system for allocation of organs for patients on the waiting list is touched on at *http://www.npr.org/blogs/health/2012/09/20/161475405/whos-next-in-line-for-a-transplant-the-answer-is-changing.*

A brilliantly written defense of the proposed new system for kidney allocation by the Committee Chairman of

OPTN/UNOS can be found at *http://blogs.law.harvard.edu/billofhealth/2012/10/03/commentary-from-optnunos-kidney-transplantation-committee-chair-john-friedewald/.*

How Will I Ever Find a Donor?

Living Kidney Donor Network: Harvey Mysel's nonprofit whose aim is to share knowledge and build the confidence to enable the life-changing benefits of living donation: *www.lkdn.org*

Paired Donationss and National Registries: Should I Be Personally Involved?

http://www.youtube.com/watch?v=eiYPDnlfN3Q

A brief but comprehensive YouTube video from Johns Hopkins on paired donation

http://www.youtube.com/watch?v=VszbcpVzz_A

Another excellent YouTube video from Duke on paired donation

National Kidney Registry: a nonprofit dedicated to increasing the quality, timeliness, and number of living donor transplants, significant registry of potential donors, and the leader in paired exchange chains amplifying the value and benefit of altruistic donation: *www.kidneyregistry.org*

The UNOS sponsored federal program: *http://communication.unos.org/2012/02/everything-you-wanted-to-know-about-the-optn-kidney-paired-donation-program/* and click on Kidney Paired Donation.

Other programs that facilitate matching between donors and recipients (registration fees may be involved):

Life Renewal: an organization that is a comprehensive resource for kidney donors and their recipients, with special attention given to the Jewish community: *www.life-renewal.org*

Another nonprofit program for matching living donors with recipients: *http://www.matchingdonor.com*

Another nonprofit program for matching living donors with recipients: *http://www.paireddonation.org*

Another nonprofit program for matching living donors with recipients: *http://www.floodsisters.org/database/index.php?link=patient*

What Does the Potential Living Donor Need to Know?

An important article from *The New England Journal of Medicine* looking at long-term follow-up of kidney donors: *http://www.nejm.org/doi/full/10.1056/NEJMoa0804883*

http://www.youtube.com/watch?v=jyovauhXEuw: Dr. Karl Womer of Johns Hopkins in a well-done brief YouTube video on what the potential kidney donor needs to know

http://www.healthnewsdigest.com/news/transplant%20 issues0/Top_10_Things_You_Should_Know_about_Organ_ Donation.shtml: A succinct review of the top ten things an organ donor should know

CNS News Katie Couric video: a capsule TV summary of living donation and the domino effect from Good Samaritan donation: *http://www.cbsnews.com/video/watch/ ?id=7042488n&tag=mncol;lst;1*

http://www.nytimes.com/2012/11/14/health/kidney-donors- given-mandatory-safeguards.html?_r=0: UNOS continuing effort to provide optimal short and long-term care for organ donors

An instructive personal narrative from an anonymous donor: *http://www.renalandurologynews.com/why-i-donated-a- kidney-anonymously/article/203527/*

Another excellent and instructive personal narrative from an author/donor who donated a kidney to her good friend: *http://www.texasmonthly.com/preview/2006-06-01/postrel*

An example of potential insurance complications for donors: *http://www.npr.org/blogs/health/2011/04/19/135537090/ give-an-organ-and-get-health-insurance-headaches*

Individual stories: the Wake Forest University baseball coach gives a kidney to one of his athletes and offers five tips to potential living donors: *http://www.kidney.org/news/ekidney/april11/CoachTomWalter_April11.cfm*

Individual stories: Miles McPherson, former NFL player and founding pastor of the Rock congregation in San Diego exhorts us to "Do Something: Make Your Life Count": *http://www.alrcnewskitchen.com/eblast/others/091007_miles-mcpherson.htm*

http://www.livingdonorassistance.org: A website providing information on federal assistance for those wanting to donate an organ but unable to because of financial constraints

The Unique and Complex World of Health Insurance Coverage for Kidney Transplant Recipients and Living Kidney Donors: Do I Really Have to Get Involved?

Several resources for additional information on Medicare coverage for dialysis and kidney transplant patients: *http://www.medicare.gov*, and type in kidney transplant

What will Post-Operative Immunosuppression and My Daily Pill Regimen Be Like?

Should I Be Considering My International Options for Transplant?

An example of transplant tourism: *http://www.angeleshealth.com/kidney-transplant*

Additional examples of horror stories from third world transplantation: *http://www.theepochtimes.com/n2/t/organ-harvesting-in-china*

http://www.bloomberg.com/news/2011-05-12/desperate-americans-buy-kidneys-from-peru-poor-in-fatal-trade.html

http://www.ipsnews.net/2011/05/china-click-your-kidney-away/

Finally, What Are Reasonable Expectations for My Outcome?